STRONG BONDS, STRONG IMMUNE SYSTEMS

STRONG BONDS, STRONG IMMUNE SYSTEMS

ARIA NIGHTINGALE

CONTENTS

CHAPTER 1

Introduction

In our journey through life, we often hear seemingly benign statements that carry a lifetime of anecdotal and experiential evidence. Such is the case when we consider the health benefits of strong social bonds. Behind these statements lies a profound understanding of how relationships can influence our well-being. Recent studies have shown that strong social networks can significantly reduce the risk of heart disease, comparable to healthy lifestyle choices such as consuming fruits and vegetables and regular exercise. This revelation has garnered much attention in scientific circles and public opinion alike.

The concept of fleeting rapport among associated proteins forming mutualistic bonds offers a fascinating glimpse into how evolution leverages social networks to maintain more than just mental health. This biological interplay mirrors the intricate social structures we form, highlighting the evolutionary benefits of social connections.

Reflecting on the vivid recollections of early center-based research on social structures, we see how these studies were often met with resistance and academic skepticism. However, the lessons learned from these historical scientific skirmishes have tempered modern discourse. Today, we recognize the importance of social bonds not only for mental and emotional well-being but also for physical health.

Across various faith traditions, spiritual leaders have guided their followers along a righteous path, instilling moral values and fostering personal growth. My grandmother, a religious mentor in my life and the last in line to receive spiritual enlightenment from Mahatma Gandhi, often imparted wisdom that transcended conventional beliefs. If you had asked her about the significance of social bonds, she would have gently rapped my knuckles and said, "My son, before acquiring any of those qualities, ensure you have real friends. Friends who stand by you through the valleys and peaks of life, friends who trust you with their well-being, and friends whom you can trust with yours."

Her words resonate deeply, reminding us that the health benefits of relationships extend beyond physical and mental wellness. They encompass the essence of our humanity, enriching our lives in profound and meaningful ways.

CHAPTER 2

The Impact of Relationships on Health

In today's fast-paced world, maintaining social connections might seem like a challenge, but the benefits are profoundly rewarding. Research indicates that staying socially connected can have a significant positive impact on your health, almost comparable to the negative impact of smoking. It's crucial to cultivate a network of at least half a dozen relationships, including family, coworkers, and community members (friends, and even friends of friends). People with strong social connections have a 50 percent lower risk of dying early compared to those who do not engage in meaningful social interactions.

Social communities and cultures profoundly shape behaviors and overall well-being. As Jesus once famously remarked, "In my hometown, nobody shows you any respect," highlighting the influence of social environments on individual behavior and community dynamics. A person who feels happy and supported is more likely to take good care of themselves and extend that care to others. Strong emotional connections also mean that you are less likely to engage in solitary, unhealthy behaviors, such as eating alone at a fast-food chain.

A comprehensive meta-analysis, reviewing data from 148 studies, found that social connection is associated with a 50 percent reduced risk of early death. The evidence is so compelling that simply knowing someone might be there for you can have substantial health benefits. People who remain socially engaged and maintain friendships tend to age more gracefully and resist the negative effects of aging. For instance, a study following 600 Californians over 25 years found that those who were less social had a 20 percent higher mortality rate, regardless of gender. Similar studies on the elderly reveal that a lack of strong relationships and increasing isolation can have devastating health impacts.

The impact of relationships on health is undeniable. Strong social connections contribute to longer life expectancy, better mental health, and a more resilient aging process. Cultivating and maintaining these relationships should be a priority for anyone looking to enhance their overall health and well-being.

CHAPTER 3

Physical Health Benefits of Strong Bonds

Good relationships help reduce stress, a significant health hazard. Scientifically, stress involves three components: a perceived threat, a physiological response, and a cognitive effort to manage the response. Stress elevates your heart rate, directs more blood to your muscles, and activates the fight-or-flight response. All of this consumes energy, diverting it away from vital functions like healing wounds, digestion, or combating viruses. Chronic stress weakens your immune response by disrupting the timing and synchronization of inflammation, essential for efficiently allocating resources.

Interestingly, psychologist Sarah Pressman from the University of Kansas notes that you don't even need to be fully aware of your social ties to benefit from them. Nonetheless, closer relationships—such as those with friends and immediate family—provide more potent relief than acquaintances. Having close relationships to turn to in times of heartbreak, to lend you a listening ear when you need it most, and to share joy with can potentially protect you against overeating, heart disease, flu, colds, depression, and even type 2 diabetes.

Recently, Sarah Pressman and Sheldon Cohen, a research psychologist at Carnegie Mellon University, reviewed data from 148 studies demonstrating the physical benefits of strong relationships. Their findings, published in the journal *Personality and Social Psychology Review*, revealed that people with robust social relationships have a 50% better chance of survival than those with weaker networks. This translates to a 1.5% increased chance of survival for individuals with enhanced social ties. This phenomenon is likely due to the fact that people with social ties encourage each other to engage in healthy activities, discourage unhealthy behaviors, and share valuable knowledge and experience.

In essence, the physical health benefits of strong bonds are multifaceted. Reduced stress, improved immune response, and the encouragement of healthy behaviors are just a few of the ways that strong relationships can contribute to overall well-being and longevity.

CHAPTER 4

Emotional Well-being and Relationships

When you're less sick, illness is less socially impactful, and thus your relationships' influence on your immune system is diminished. Consequently, important health outcomes depend more on your effort and attitudes rather than your relationships. However, when you're gravely ill with something dangerous, easily spread, and not well understood, others also bear the consequences. In such situations, having strong, committed, and loving relationships with your partner or family members can guide their—and the community's—attitudes, actions, and support towards nursing you back to health.

Hostility and criticism predict new health problems not merely because being around such negativity is damaging but because we tend to either avoid hostile and critical partners or react chemically with them, which can slow recovery and exacerbate issues. When your partner is critical or hostile, your body reacts with higher stress hormone levels, leading to a weakened immune system about eight hours later, effectively slowing down recovery.

In a loving, supportive, and committed relationship, why does it hurt so much when you argue or feel rejected by your long-term partner? Partly, it's because your immune system has a built-in vulnerability to social conflict and environmental stress, especially from those who matter the most to you. When your partner is kind and supportive, your immune system functions more robustly. Conversely, when your partner is hostile or critical, your immune system weakens. The fear of your partner's reaction to an argument or rejection then becomes a risk factor for new health problems.

You become vulnerable to physical problems because your emotional reactions to your long-term partner also influence how you feel and behave when you're sick or around infectious people. Consequently, new health conditions can escalate more rapidly when you become ill, and once you're ill, your recovery is slower.

CHAPTER 5

Social Support and Health

In the last year of her life, my maternal grandmother spent a lot of time with her family in the Black Hills. One night, my mother fell asleep to the sounds of her parents talking. Knowing that Mommom was sick and lonely, she went into the room to join the conversation. When she woke up the next morning, she found them asleep—my grandfather curled up in the recliner with my grandmother's head resting on his lap. My mother realized they had stayed awake, talking through the night. This personal care provided by my grandfather was essential for my grandmother's well-being. Despite being in the late stages of cancer, she never felt unloved or unsupported. This story beautifully illustrates the power of social support in action, offering protection against infectious germs and other health risks we face.

Our immune systems are designed to keep us safe, even in the face of stress, be it from chronic illness, food scarcity, or other challenges. One of the most crucial sources of social support comes from close personal relationships—whether with friends or spouses. Research consistently shows that a network of strong relationships has beneficial effects on people's lives. For instance, when students on a waiting list for counseling had strong ties to friends and neighbors, they showed significant improvement without formal help. Conversely, chronic loneliness can lead to weakened immune systems, inflamed tissues, and increased risk of heart disease due to stress.

In essence, social support is vital for our overall health and well-being. It not only helps us cope with physical illnesses but also bolsters our emotional resilience. Building and maintaining strong relationships is essential for navigating life's challenges and enhancing our quality of life.

CHAPTER 6

Relationship Quality and Immune System

My hypothesis—that relationship quality is tied to immune function—is supported by several studies. In one notable study, participants developed small blisters on the backs of their arms to measure how quickly their bodies would heal, and then engaged in significant conversations with their partners. When the partner was available before the blistering procedure, participants talked for longer. Those who felt better about their relationships had quicker healing times once the blister was created. Kaplan-Meier curves suggest that participants in high-quality relationships were twice as likely to have healed after 32 days compared to those in low-quality relationships. In fewer than nine days, 82% of high-quality relationship participants had healed, compared to only 46% of their low-quality peers. The age of the participants was relatively balanced, with high-quality relationship participants averaging 43.9 years old, and low-quality participants averaging 44.9 years old. This result indicates that participants with high relationship quality expected more social support, leading to quicker and healthier recovery.

People thrive when they have strong, positive relationships, whether romantic, friendly, or familial. We are innately social creatures, with the drive to connect hardwired into our DNA. But what is the science behind the benefits of strong bonds? How exactly do relationships improve health? In a recent scientific paper, I identified one mechanism linking strong relationships to health: the immune system. I propose that high relationship quality—characterized by love, support, and warmth—may help people experience an improved immune system, leading to better physical health. After all, humans evolved to be more social than any other primates, making relationships essential for good health. Our immune system adapted to respond quickly to insults, such as viruses, and having a ready response against infection allowed our ancestors to recover more easily from illnesses.

CHAPTER 7

The Role of Communication in Health

Supportive communication styles can foster not only psychological health but physical well-being as well. Numerous studies have supported this idea. For instance, recent research on normative populations found that engaging in even a few close conversations towards the end of the day predicted better self-reported health the next day. Similar links have been uncovered in various health-update studies.

My own research has focused on the physiological benefits of everyday supportive communication within long-term committed relationships. These investigations have shown that having a number of close conversations where one feels encouraged and loved can reduce everyday stress on both physical and psychological levels.

Close relationships offer numerous opportunities for the communication of social and emotional support. Recently, researchers have started to examine the extent to which this type of communication can also promote physical health and well-being. It is now recognized that social support operates in two fashions—helpful and potentially harmful. When individuals engage in supportive interactions and when social circle members are mutually supportive, they can experience a reduction in stress and activation of the parasympathetic branch of the autonomic nervous system. Conversely, unsupportive behavior and conflict can elevate salivary cortisol levels, negatively impacting the health and well-being of individuals and social networks.

Engaging in supportive communication fosters an environment where stress is reduced, and the body's natural healing processes are enhanced. This highlights the importance of positive, supportive interactions in maintaining and improving overall health.

CHAPTER 8

Building and Maintaining Strong Bonds

To fully reap the immunoprotective benefits, relationships need to be both strong and long-lasting. Building and maintaining such bonds takes effort and isn't as straightforward as simple friendships or acquaintanceships. Good, strong relationships take time to develop and can often evolve from mutual productive working experiences, sharing discussion groups, conversation clubs, and engaging in lengthy behavioral and personal discussions. In such environments, personal visions can be mutually elaborated, and intellectual and ambitious projects can be designed together. These collaborations help create and reinforce consistently renewing forces in friendships, orchestrated around the idea that nothing beneficial is achieved without sound goals, sensible demands, and healthy needs ratios.

Having strong, nurturing relationships is fundamental to our happiness and emotional health. A positive emotional atmosphere can enhance our health, just as negative emotions can suppress the functioning of the immune system. Certain aspects of relationships can help improve our immune functioning. For instance, studies on healthy college students and older adults engaged in supportive telephone conversations have shown increased immune response in both groups. Self-disclosures, rather than chat content, were associated with improved immune profiles. Additionally, studies have noted a link between social isolation and compromised immune response in depressed individuals.

In one study focusing on women with breast cancer, having a support partner from the initial acceptance of the diagnosis through the first major treatment was associated with reduced levels of infectious illness for the patients but not for their support partners. This highlights the profound impact of having a dedicated support system during challenging times.

Building and maintaining strong bonds requires dedication and effort, but the benefits are immense. Strong relationships not only enhance our emotional well-being but also provide critical support for our physical health. They foster resilience, offer protection against various health risks, and contribute to a happier, healthier life.

CHAPTER 9

Strategies for Strengthening Relationships

There is no single solution to help people become less lonely and more connected. Loneliness is a complex condition influenced by various factors, including psychological health, mental health, physical health, and work, family, and community conditions. Bringing isolated people together in support groups, classes, or other settings so they can learn from others' experiences is a key starting point. Training individuals to develop better and more satisfying relationships can provide them with tools to end isolation. Additionally, access to medical care for those coping with challenging life circumstances can help restore strength and vitality when it seems impossible. To facilitate finding thought-provoking and supportive friends, our social institutions must take steps to reduce poverty and improve the quality of education. Embracing a bit of Groucho Marx's non-judgmental, fun-loving, Marx Brothers camaraderie can inspire and guide changes that will help pull people out of their solitude and foster meaningful connections.

Research shows that while we cannot change our friends exactly, we can spend more time with good friends and strengthen bonds within our existing social networks. For example, Shauna Gray, PhD, and colleagues from Arizona State University found that women who increased interactions with friends over a nine-month period had stronger immune responses across various branches of the immune system. Furthermore, people with strong and varied social networks were four times more likely to survive a serious illness than those without such connections.

Strengthening relationships involves several strategies:

1. **Organize Social Gatherings**: Plan regular get-togethers, such as dinner parties, game nights, or outdoor activities, to foster closeness and create lasting memories.
2. **Join Clubs or Groups**: Engage in clubs, classes, or community groups that align with your interests to meet like-minded individuals and build new friendships.
3. **Practice Active Listening**: Show genuine interest in others by listening actively, asking questions, and offering support during conversations.
4. **Express Appreciation**: Regularly express gratitude and appreciation for the people in your life to strengthen emotional bonds.
5. **Be Supportive**: Offer help and support during difficult times and celebrate successes to build trust and deepen relationships.
6. **Stay Connected**: Make an effort to stay in touch with friends and family through phone calls, messages, or social media, even when life gets busy.
7. **Address Conflicts**: Tackle conflicts head-on with open communication and a willingness to understand the other person's perspective.

By adopting these strategies, we can create and maintain strong, nurturing relationships that enhance our overall well-being and provide a robust support network during life's challenges.

CHAPTER 10

Conclusion

The results indicate that lifestyle interventions can reduce illness more effectively than usual care. However, these interventions have only a slight influence when addressing the loneliness of older individuals. We suggest that older adults may need specific interventions to tackle loneliness, as it can be more challenging to overcome when they are in poor physical health and living alone. Seriously lonely older adults should be recognized and targeted as an important group with both mental and physical health issues. Future studies should examine the immunologic and endocrinologic functions in lonely older individuals to better understand and address their needs. Enhancing interpersonal connections appears to be a crucial component in increasing the benefits of existing lifestyle care services for older people.

This chapter has focused on the close relationships in our lives for a good reason. Solid empirical evidence shows that the warmth and emotional support from our partners, families, and friends are significant protective factors for our health. There is strong evidence that individuals who feel preference and support from others are happier and have fewer physical and emotional health problems. Building and maintaining strong relationships can profoundly impact our overall well-being, making it essential to prioritize these connections in our lives.